ROBERT TACKETT

THE ABC'S OF FIRST AID STEPS FOR YOUNG ADULTS

AuthorHouse™
1663 Liberty Drive
Bloomington, IN 47403
www.authorhouse.com
Phone: 1 (833) 262-8899

This book is printed on acid-free paper.

ISBN: 978-1-7283-6721-7 (sc)
ISBN: 978-1-7283-6722-4 (e)

Library of Congress Control Number: 2020913191

Print information available on the last page.

Published by AuthorHouse 07/25/2020

authorHOUSE®

THE ABC'S OF FIRST AID STEPS FOR YOUNG ADULTS

Written by Robert Tackett

LOOK FOR OUR OTHER BOOKS COMING SOON:

The ABC's of Self Defense for kids and young adults

The ABC's of Eating Healthy for kids and young adults

The Adventure Club: First Year

The Adventure Club: 2nd Year

The Adventure Club: Abroad

On the Razor's Edge: Prequel to the Adventure Club Series

———◆•◆•◆———

This book is dedicated to my mother, Dolores.
The most beautiful soul I have ever known.

———◆•◆•◆———

This book has been written for older children ages 12 to 17. Younger children and teenagers often find themselves the first responders until an adult can be located and arrives. This book is designed to be read and discussed with parents or teachers in order to promote knowledge and understanding of what order their actions should be taken. It is important to remember that this book is not intended to be a standalone book. Rather a supplemental tool to help young adults memorize a practical and systematic approach to helping perform the steps for first aid. Read, practice and memorize these easy to learn C-A-B-Cs.

There are many agencies already in place which do a great job of teaching, training and providing much needed first aid "How to" training books and videos for adults. Visit their websites for more information on how to treat specific injuries (This would be the Fix portion of this book).

    American Red Cross

    American Heart Association

    Medic One

    National Safety Council

    American Safety and Health Institute

PREFACE

If you can read on your own and understand what you read, this book can help you help others. If you can memorize the ABCs and you have some good detective skills, this book is for you. Try to do the first aid steps in order. If you forget which step you are on, it's ok, don't panic. Just start over at "A" and continue helping all the way through "M". The alphabet starts with the letter "A". But when it comes to first aid, the first letter is always "C". After reading this book, I am sure you will understand why. This book aims to bridge the gap between performing a first aid skill and the order in which it should be performed. Let's get these younger adults ready to assist in first aid response by following simple, easy to memorize steps.

These steps to the ABCs of first aid are in an easy to memorize order. These steps will not change. C, A through M will help you actually help someone who needs it. N through Z is all about what you can do to be prepared for an emergency. Sometimes we get overwhelmed when an emergency occurs. Practice and Preparation is the key to success.

This book is not designed to be read like an adventure story. It is intended to be read with an adult, a section at a time, think about that section, ask questions, discuss it, practice it and then cover the next section. By learning this simple method of prioritizing the steps for first aid, you can confidently help others in a very precise and smooth manner. These steps can be applied to any emergency situation. Incidentally, you will understand when you can skip over a letter because it is obvious that letter is not an issue for that specific emergency. The more you practice these steps in order, the better prepared you will be to help during an emergency. Have fun learning!

It could happen scenario:

You and your younger sister are outside in the backyard playing badminton while your father is up on a ladder cleaning leaves out of the gutter. You hear him yell "Oh no"! You turn to see the ladder sliding down the side of the house and your father is dangling from the gutter with one hand. The gutter gives way and you see your father fall. You quickly close your eyes. When you open them, you see your father laying on his side and he isn't moving. You quickly run to his side and…

The first letter in the ABCs of first aid is always "**C**". If you notice someone who might need help, use your detective skills to "C" the big picture. The 4 C's to help you see the big picture are **Check, Call, Care and Control**.

Check-Check the area to make sure it is safe to be there. Check how many injured people need help, give a good guess. This should take just a moment. Check injured person(s) for responsiveness (Hey, can you hear me? Are you ok?) to make sure they really need or want help. Sometimes people do not want help. Try to figure what caused the injury(s) so you can avoid it or get the right person to fix it. Based upon what you see, hear and smell-What injuries do you think the person has?

Call-Call for help. Call an adult or maybe even Call 9-1-1 before you even try to help the injured person(s). This is the first Call. When you talk to an adult or when the dispatcher answers your phone call, tell them-

_____Your name
_____Where you and the injured person are
_____How many people are hurt
_____The kind of injury you see
_____Are any dangerous situations involved
_____Is anything special needed

Decide if you want to make the call for help before you start helping the injured person. This way you can help them while the ambulance is already on it's way. Call for or ask those people around you for additional resources. Ask for: More people, first aid kit, AED, stretcher, blanket, traffic control, gas company, water company, electric company, animal control, etc. Should take a minute or 2.

Care-Protect yourself (Put on gloves if you have them) then you can Care for the injured person. Obtain Consent first from the injured. (You're bleeding. Can I help you?). You can even give the injured person the first aid equipment and maybe they can do it themselves without you touching them. Following the letters- A through G should take less than 10 minutes to "Fix" any problems as long as you have all the tools you need. Now you are ready for the rest of the ABCs, H through M.

Control-Control what you can control. Remember to ask others to help control the scene: They can help direct traffic, meet the ambulance and bring them to you, help move a person, bring a first aid kit, etc. Also, Control any major bleeding. This is the same as applying direct pressure, meaning to squeeze the bleeding area tightly with a clean bandage, towel, shirt etc. For about 5 minutes then tie it tight-About 1 finger tight. Applying a tourniquet is a special way to control major bleeding from an arm or leg, but not always recommended if you can get to the hospital quickly. Tourniquets are serious business and not to be taken lightly. This topic needs a long, serious discussion with an adult.

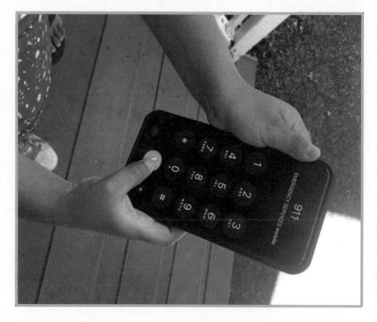

Scenario:

You and your friend are riding your bikes to Grandmother's house. When you arrive, you knock on the front door and no one answered. You try the doorknob and discover it is unlocked. You open the door, calling for your grandmother. Looking into the house you can see the kitchen. The oven door is open and now you can smell gas in the house. Begin **C4** now. **Check** the scene to ensure it is safe to be there. You see your Grandmother staggering towards you. She is covering her mouth with a dishtowel. You call for your Grandmother. You wisely decide not to enter, but you encourage her to follow your voice and she makes it to you. You know it is not safe to be in or around a house which may have a gas leak. You and your friend **Care** for her by helping her out of the house and into the fresh air. Your grandmother is coughing uncontrollably. You and your friend help her walk to the neighbor's house. Enroute, you ask if anyone else is in the house. Grandmother says "No. No one else is there". You relax a little. You sit her on the steps of the neighbor's house and ask your friend to go knock on the door (**Control**). No one is home. You send him to check another house to **Call** for help. Focusing on Grandmother, you begin the **ABC**'s of first aid. She is coughing less now so her **Airway** is intact. She can talk better now, her **Breathing** isn't the best, but it is improving. You quickly check her over to make sure she isn't bleeding anywhere. You don't notice any bleeding, so her **Circulation** must be intact. You ask her how she feels. She says her chest hurts from the coughing and she has a horrible headache. These are her **Disabilities**. You quickly ask her if everything else is ok: Her arms and hands. Her legs and knees. She adds that her fingers are tingling. Since there is no injury needing to be **Exposed**, you focus on **Fixing** her disabilities. Your friend arrives with a neighbor and a cell phone. They hand you the phone and it's 9-1-1. You state "This is _____ I am at _____with my grandmother. We found her in her home and I think it has a gas leak. She was by herself. She is having chest pain and a bad headache. We need someone to turn off the gas in the house and come and help her". The EMS dispatcher tells you someone

4

is on the way. You wisely decide not to **Go** to the ER, but to wait for the ambulance. The EMS dispatcher tells you to make your grandmother comfortable in order to **Halt** any complications from shock. You lay her back a little so she can breathe easier. You begin to gather **Information** which may be useful to the medics.

You ask your grandmother, "What happened"?
She says she was preheating the oven and went to get the ingredients for a cake she was about to bake and she forgot she had left the oven door down.
You ask if she has any allergies and she replied, "No". She doesn't.
You ask if she is taking any medications, vitamins or supplements.
She states, "Just multivitamins once a day and my insulin".
You ask about any medical conditions.
She says, "Just my diabetes, but it is well controlled".
You ask about the last time she ate or drank anything and she replies, "It was breakfast, a couple hours ago. Eggs and bacon with coffee".
"Good job". You tell her. "Just relax and breathe normal. Help is on the way". As if on cue, you can hear the sound of the firetruck sirens getting louder.

You quickly try to **Jot** down her vital signs, but since you don't have a pen and paper you tell your friend to remember them. Your Grandmother is breathing about 18 times a minute. Her pulse is about 90 times a minute. Her skin feels clammy (sweaty) and she looks very pale. The neighbor is waiting for the firetruck at the sidewalk. As the firetruck rolls up, the neighbor waves them over and points in your direction. You check your Grandmother and make sure she is still comfortable and still breathing. This is **Keeping** things right and keeping things tight.

The first rescuer walks up to you with a first aid bag over one shoulder and asks "What's going on"? You **Let them know** your Grandmother's house may have a gas leak and you point to her home. He radios to his crew and you can see firemen and firewomen putting on their masks and helmets. They begin walking towards your grandmother's house. You turn back to your grandmother who seems to be embarrassed as she realizes she is the center of all the commotion. The fireman kneels down to begin examining your grandmother. You explain to the fireman everything you know and did. This is the **Medical hand off.** Now you can relax and catch your breath. The fireman puts your grandmother on some oxygen, using a clear, see-through mask attached to a bag which inflates and deflates with each breath your grandmother takes. He continues to examine your grandmother and asks more questions. A few minutes later, the fire crew walks back to their truck. One of the fire guys comes over and while he is taking off his helmet and mask he says,

"Your grandmother is extremely lucky that you two got here when you did. The pilot light for the oven must have gone out for some reason. We opened all the windows to get fresh air in and let the gas out. Don't go back there for a few hours".

The first Rescuer asks, "Is there someone we can call to come and pick everyone up"?

Before answering, your Grandmother gives you a great big hug.

Now, let's get to it! After you have considered the C4 concepts you can now focus on the injured person(s).

A – Airway Is it open?

Make sure they can keep their airway open. If they cannot keep their airway open on their own, you may have to help them – Take 10 seconds or less to check: If the injured person is talking or crying, then their airway is open and they are probably breathing.

If you are not sure if the person is breathing:

Look, Listen and Feel

Discuss ways to keep airways open:

Head tilt / Chin Lift

Make sure their airway stays open:

Keep them talking

If you have to, hold their head and neck in such a way that their airway doesn't close

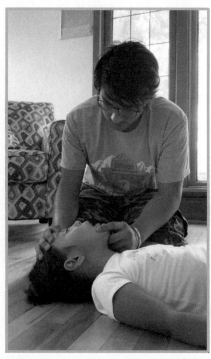

B – Breathing Is it good enough?

Make sure the injured person(s) are breathing enough – Take less than 10 seconds to check

Get your face close to theirs and Look, Listen and Feel with 1 easy movement.

Look for the rise and fall of their chest

Listen for them to be breathing

Feel for air coming from their nose and mouth with your cheek

Look at their face. Is their face normal color?

Blue? Red? Splotchy? Grey/Ashen?

Does their breathing sound different than yours? Are they choking?

Do the Heimlich maneuver, modified abdominal thrusts or modified chest thrusts, if you are properly trained.

If they are not breathing enough-Do something

Consider CPR

Consider rescue breathing

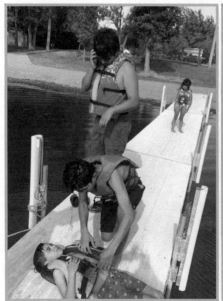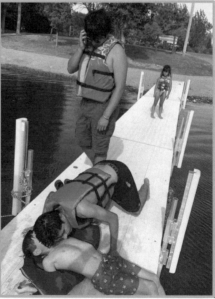

C – Circulation Is their heart beating enough to keep them alive?

If they are talking, crying, etc. They probably have a good pulse and you can skip this part. If they are not moving or not responding you might want to check their pulse:

Check for a pulse-Do not count it, just check to make sure they have a pulse. Touch the side of their neck with your 2 fingers. Do you feel their heart beat? Take less than 10 seconds to check. If they don't have a pulse, consider doing CPR (cardiopulmonary resuscitation), if you have been properly trained.

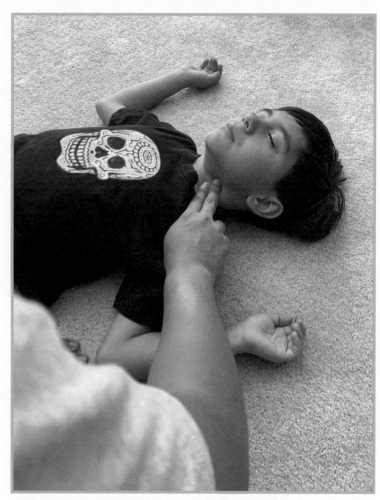

If you choose not to do CPR:

Is anyone available who can?

Is there an AED nearby? Many public places have AEDs on site: Malls, theatres, large companies, large stores, libraries, schools, etc.

Check their skin:

Skin is warm/normal/dry?

Skin is cool/clammy or hot/dry to the touch?

D – Disability What is the main problem?

> Ask the injured person what happened? Ask them where it hurts? Use your detective skills – Maybe they cannot speak (too young, mute, etc.). Maybe they do not speak your language.
> Try to figure out what their main problem is.

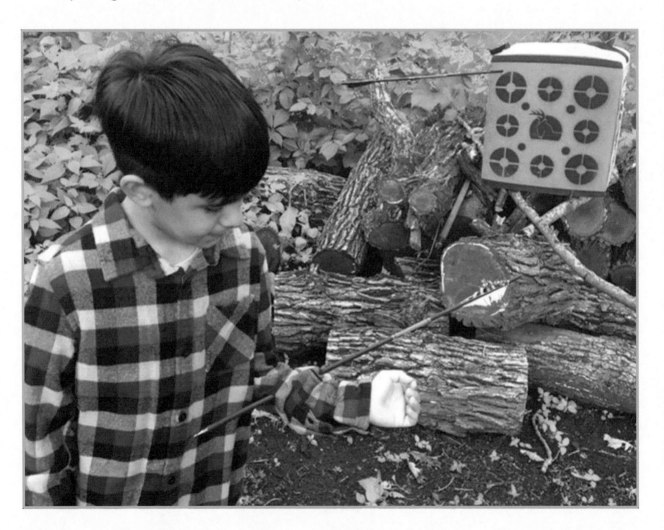

E – Expose and Examine Get a good look at the injury. Say the problem out loud.

Focus on where they say it hurts. Expose the area, but do not cause further harm.
It takes a lot of practice. Examine the injury, but be gentle.
Roll up a sleeve or pant leg
Take off a shoe and sock
Remove a jacket

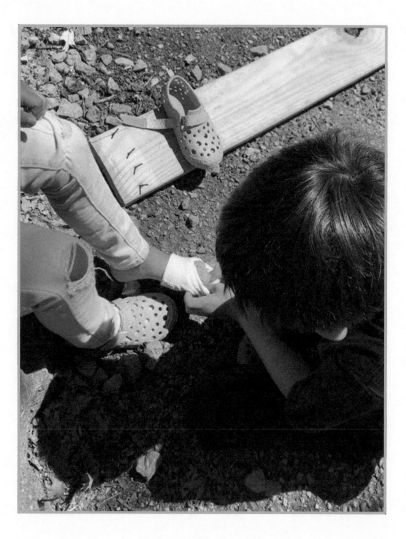

F – Fix the problem Say out loud what you are doing.

This helps you focus on what you are doing and also helps reassure the injured person that you are helping. Fix any problems as you find them.

1. Clean minor wounds: Use soap and water, apply antibiotic ointments, apply covering bandage
2. Bleeding cuts: Press directly on the cut to stop or slow down the bleeding (Also called applying direct pressure). Use a clean bandage if you have one available.
Apply bandages – Usually 1 or 2 fingers tight
3. Dizziness: Sit them down or lay them down
4. Smash, crush, Bruises and twisted joints: Try to keep it still, don't move it too much, Put on padded splints – Not to tight, just tight enough to keep it still
Use ice packs – Don't freeze the skin, cool down the muscle
5. Minor Burns: Redness with maybe some small blistering area, Run cold water over the area for 10 minutes
6. Allergic reaction: Get them their medication so they can take it. Stay focused on their airway remaining open
7. Something gets in your eye(s): Rinse eye(s) for at least 15 minutes with cool, clean water

Some problems you cannot fix. You will need to get someone who can fix them: Adult, paramedic, fireman, nurse or a doctor. For example:
Asthma, breathing problems or choking
Earache
Headache
Vomiting
Uncontrollable bleeding
Chest Pain
Unconscious-Can't wake them up

Think about what you need to do. Ask: What is the best way to fix the problem with the resources and time I have available?

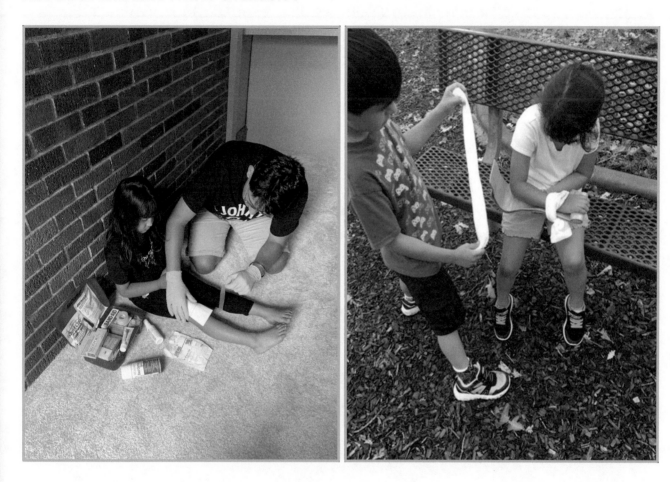

G – Go or Stay Make a decision.

Decide -If you should take the injured person to a hospital on your own
      -Go somewhere it is easier to meet an ambulance or
      -Wait where you are for an ambulance to come to you
Just make a decision and go with that. If your decision is to move someone, be very careful and try not to cause any further injuries.

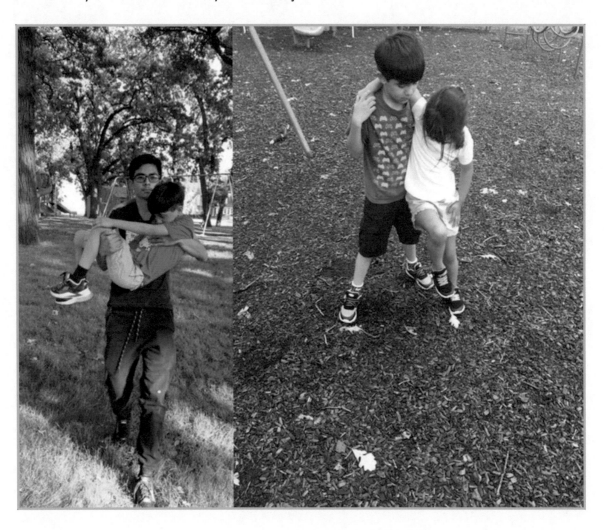

Scenario:

You are babysitting your cousins. They are 3 and 5 years old. You are watching tv in the living room while they are upstairs in their bedroom asleep, or so you thought. You hear a loud thump from upstairs. You go to investigate. You check on the kids by looking through the open door. This begins **C4. Check**ing for any hazards, the area looks safe enough to enter. You Call out for the kids in a quiet voice.

You see one of the cousins, the youngest, on the floor having what appears to be a seizure. You may even feel helpless. You remember your uncle telling you about seizures last year. You quickly begin to **Control** the scene by making sure there is nothing sharp or hard that can cause injury, in case your cousin hits it while having this seizure. This is the first step to **Care** for your cousin. You wake up the older cousin and have them go get the house phone. You are closely watching the seizure go through its motions. It seems very scary. Your cousin arrives with the phone. You quickly **Call** your aunt and uncle to tell them what's happening. They reassure you that it is going to be ok. They are on their way back home. You hang up as the seizure has run it's course. You get down close to your little cousin and check the **Airway** to make sure he is positioned in such a way that his airway stays open. You look, listen and feel for **Breathing.** He is. You give him a good "Once over" (Checking to ensure his **Circulation** is intact) to ensure he isn't bleeding anywhere and you notice he is starting to bleed from his nose. You lay your cousin on his side and ask your other cousin to get a towel for the bleeding. As the little guy starts to wake up, you know he will be scared, especially when he sees the blood from his nose. You ask him how he feels and he responds slowly that he is scared and tired, very tired. This is checking him for a **Disability.** The disabilities you have noticed are seizure, nose bleed, and fatigue, so far. You sit him up in your lap and lean him forward while you pinch the bridge of his nose to help stop the bleeding. You are ready to lay him back down if a seizure starts again. There is no injury you need to **Expose** at this time. You are **Fixing** one of the problems by controlling the nose bleed and ensuring the blood doesn't go down the back of the throat. You decide not to **Go** anywhere and stay where you are, upstairs in the bedroom waiting for your aunt and uncle. You cover your little cousin with a sheet to **Halt** any shock symptoms, being very careful not to cover his neck or face. The older cousin wants to go downstairs to watch cartoons, but you tell him that you need him to stay with you in case you need more help. You review the **Information** that you have: 3-year-old cousin with a history of seizures. No allergies that you know of. You remember that he does take a medication every day to help prevent seizures. They ate some pizza and had juice at 6pm before going to bed at 9pm. You tell your older cousin to get a piece of paper and a pen. You **Jot** down the vital signs as you check them. Breathing 20 times a minute. Pulse is 90 times a minute. Skin is warm and dry. You get your little cousin cleaned up with a damp towel and he starts to fall asleep. The nose bleed has stopped so you lay him down on his side covered with the sheet. You sit down next to him, **Keep**ing things right and keeping things tight. You hear your aunt and uncle come in the front door. They make it upstairs to find you watching over their child. You **Let** them know everything that transpired (happened). They decide a **Medical Hand off** is not needed and they will closely monitor their child's condition and discuss it with their pediatrician in the morning. You need a raise!

H - Halt the Shock Halfway finished. The Hard part is over

Treat everyone for Shock

      Remain calm, even if you are scared or nervous
      If it's cold out-warm them up
      If it's hot out-cool them down
      Elevate the feet, if the feet and legs are not injured
      Make them comfortable
            Have them sit up if it helps them breath
            Loosen up all restrictive (tight) clothing
      Do not let injured people eat or drink anything
      If they may vomit, consider laying them on their side with one hand under their head.

Remember, Shock is a lot like Love-There are varying degrees of Love, i.e. Infatuation, puppy love, a crush, true love, etc. Lots of things can cause you to feel like you are in love, i.e. dopamine, oxytocin, euphoria, etc.

Shock also has varying degrees, i.e. mild, moderate, severe and irreversible. Likewise, there are lots of things can cause a person to suffer from Shock, i.e. hypovolemia, neurogenic, toxic, cardiogenic, anaphylactic, etc.

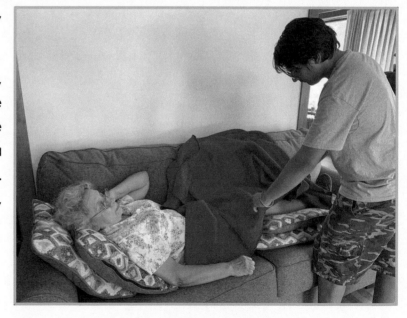

I - Information gathering

Gather important information – From the injured person(s) or from any witnesses. What's their name and age? Is there anyone you can call for them?

> S-Statement of what happened?
> A-Any allergies? Ask about medical alert tags/bracelets. Look for them
> M-Medications? Ask them if they have any medications on them and do they need help taking it. Have they taken any medications, supplements or drugs recently?
> P-Pertinent medical history? Any recent medical conditions? Like surgeries, diabetes, etc.
> L-Last time they ate or drank. What was it? How much?

J – Jot down their Vital Signs You should always have a pen and paper.

Check vital signs at least twice-5 to 10 minutes apart – Are they improving?

> Pulse: Count it now for 1 full minute
> Breathing: Count it now for 1 full minute
> Skin: Touch and look at their skin. Check for these 3 things-
> > Color-Red, pink, blue, splotchy, pale, grey/ashen
> > Condition-Dry, clammy, sweaty
> > Temperature-Hot or cool

K – Keep things right, keep things tight

Check everything you did over again

      Airway, Breathing, Circulation
      Bleeding is controlled
      Bandages are still working
      Splints are still tight
      Cold packs are working and not freezing the skin
      Any Medications they took are working

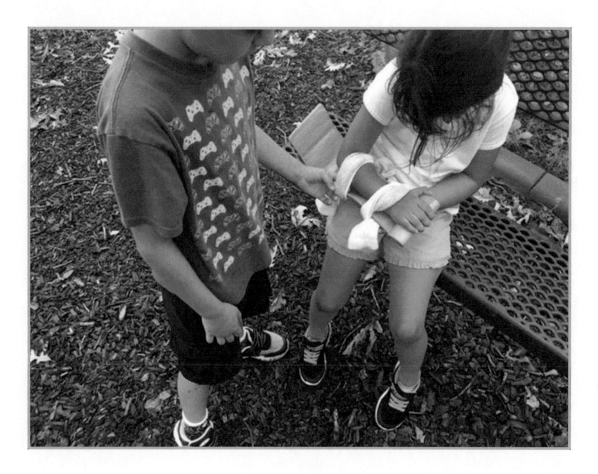

L – Let others know Don't keep any secrets. Tell them everything This is the 2nd call.

Call the hospital or tell the ambulance crew everything you did to help. Also let them know when the injured person will get there.
Give them the information you gathered (SAMPL, Vital Signs)
Call their family members

M – Medical Hand Off

Turn over the injured person to someone more trained than yourself. i.e.an adult, medics, nurses, doctors, etc. Tell them everything. Paint them a picture (describe and explain) of what has been going on.
You are halfway through the alphabet of ABCs for First Aid. C-A-B-C-D-E-F-G-H-I-J-K-L-M is the hard part. This is the part where you physically take direct action.
The rest of the alphabet N-O-P-Q-R-S-T-U-V-W-X-Y-Z is all about knowledge and being prepared. Relax now and remember to breathe.

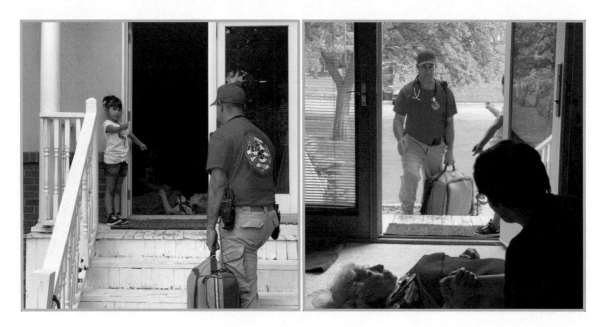

N – Not going to happen to me. Never let it happen again

Understand that the world is not fair and bad things are going to happen to good people. Stay focused and do the best you can.
Learn from the past and prepare yourself and your loved ones. Correct any unsafe issues at home to prevent them from hurting others

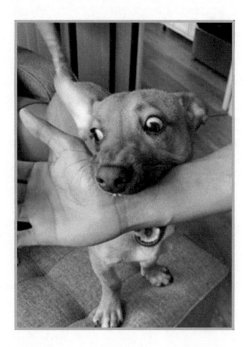

O – Open your mind. Be Observant and Objective.

Remember-New techniques and medications are being designed and improved upon all the time. Stay up to date with regular training and practice.
Be Observant and recognize potentially dangerous situations before anyone gets hurt. This takes a very special kind of skill.
Recognizing that danger and taking precautions to prevent injuries takes a very special kind of person. Be that person.

P – Planning, Preparation, Practice and Prevention Putting it all together.

Planning-Plan what to do for different emergencies. i.e. fire, gas leak, someone fell out of a tree, etc.

Preparation-Know where your resources are. i.e. first aid kit, blankets, gloves, maps, etc.

Practice-Practice each first aid skill. i.e. applying a bandage, applying a splint, etc.

Prevention-Keep chemicals out of the reach of children, put safety locks on cupboards and safety caps on outlets, etc. Keep in mind that emergencies can be overwhelming. We will forget somethings and we will do things out of order, don't panic or become frustrated, just do your best to help and try not to cause any further harm. As you find yourself helping others, you will gain experience and you will get better and better at it. This is why they call it "Practicing medicine".

Where are your fire extinguishers located in your home?

> Place extinguishers in easy to find/view locations. Inspect fire extinguishers weekly for the arrow to be in the green (meaning the fire extinguisher is still pressurized and charged.
>
> PASS: Pull the pin, Aim the nozzle at the base of the fire, Squeeze the trigger, Sweep the spray from side to side.
>
> Does your family have different types of fire extinguishers? Type A, type, B, type C, type A-B-C

What are the different types of fire extinguishers for?

Where does your family keep the first aid kit? Where in the home? Where in the vehicle?

How often do you check your smoke and carbon monoxide alarms? Every 6 months?

When your family goes on an outing, do you have a quick Safety Briefing before leaving?

Where you are going?

What route will you be taking?

How long you will be gone?

What are your main means to communicate? Cell phones, radios.

Where is the closest medical center?

Where are the important items located? Is the first aid kit in the trunk or a backpack?

Where are the flashlights? Do they work? What about light sticks or flares? Do we need wet weather gear? Cold weather gear?

Plan your equipment and supplies based upon your activity, weather and time of year.

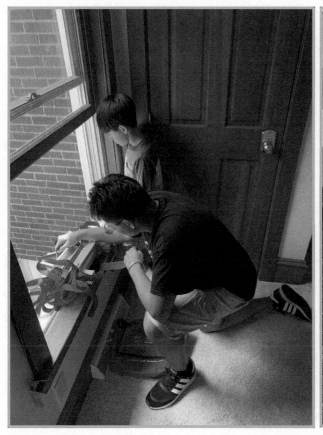
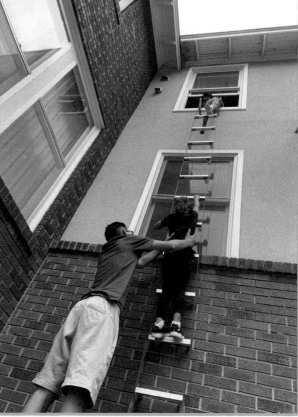

Q – Question any and all pain! Ask these questions:

 O-Onset. When did the pain begin?
 P-Provokes. What causes the pain to worsen or get better?
 Q-Quality. What kind (type) of pain is it? Describe it: Sharp, dull, deep, achy?
 R-Radiating. Does the pain start somewhere and go somewhere else?
 S-Severity. How bad is the pain? On a scale of 1 to 10, 10 being the worst pain ever!
 T-Time. When did the pain begin?

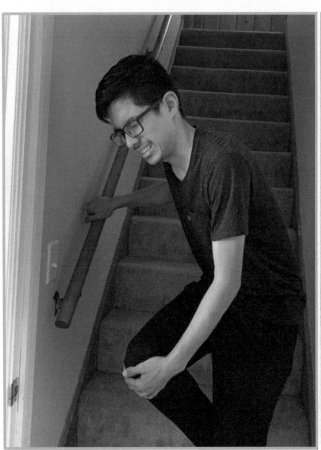
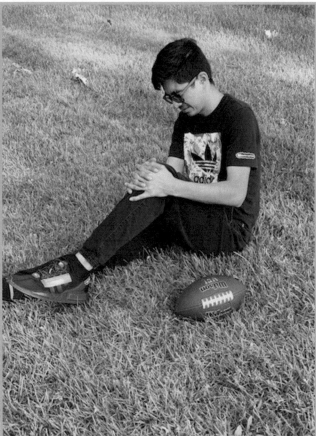

R – Recognize what is an emergency and what isn't.

Each of these conditions need to be thoroughly explained by an adult in detail to better understand them. You can also learn more about these types of medical complications by researching them using some of the companies mentioned in the beginning of this book.

Emergency	Not an emergency
Seizure that's unexpected	Normal Seizure lasting less than 5 minutes
Heart attack	Short of breath for less than 1 minute
Fractures and dislocations	Joint sprains and muscle strains
Stroke	Lumps, bumps and bruises
Asthma and other breathing problems	Coughing
Allergic reactions	Vomiting
Severe bleeding	Scrapes, splinters and cuts
Unconscious person	Sleeping or tired
Burns bigger than your hand	Minor burns and minor sunburns
Eye injuries	Dust in your eyes
Poisoning	Diarrhea, unless it has blood in it!
Choking on food or objects	Choking while drinking liquids
Animal bite: Dog, snake, zombie	Scratches and stings
Dehydrated	Thirsty
Malnourished	Hungry

S – Start doing something: Follow the steps C4 and A thru M.

Don't be afraid to act. There is always something you can do to help. Always protect yourself if you are going to help someone you don't know.

If you are unsure of how to help, call for an ambulance. Give them the first aid supplies and let them help themselves.

What is the EMS number for your area? 9-1-1, 1-1-2, 9-9-9, 9-2-2, etc.

T2 – Talk about things before an emergency happens and also **Talk** about it afterwards with your family and friends.

Before:	Do any close friends or family members have a condition which is contagious?
	Example: Covid 19/Corona Virus, Cold, Flu, Hepatitis, HIV, Tuberculosis, etc.
	Do any close friends or family members have a medical condition you may have to help with?
	Example: Seizures, Colostomy/Stoma bag, Diabetes, Allergies, etc.
After:	Tell someone what you thought was going on
	Talk about what was going through your mind
	Now that you think about it-What could have been done better?
Remember:	Some people do not want others to know about their medical issues. Respect their decision.
	With that understanding, protect yourself from possible contagious illnesses.

U – Understand the possible hazards you may face.

   Are any rattlesnakes in your neighborhood?
   Does diabetes run in your family?
   Do you have little toddlers/children in the house?
   Is there a swimming pool/creek/river/lake close by?
   Does the house have any bad electrical wiring?
   Are you going out on a boat? Reach, Throw, Don't go!
   "Knowing is half the battle". -G. I. Joe

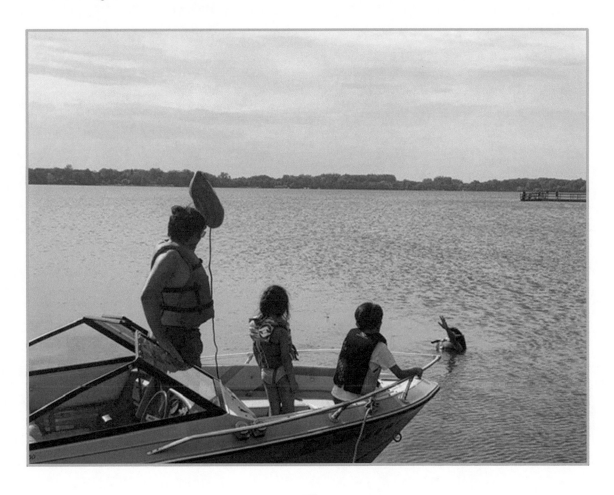

V – Verify your stuff regularly

Verify you are up to date:

Immunizations-Ask your family members about your shots
Training – Most agencies recommend training every 2 years
First aid kits-House, car and backpack. Check monthly
Medications-Liquids, injections, creams, and pills. Check yearly
Flashlights work-Kitchen, garage, car, bedrooms. Check weekly
Fire extinguishers are ready-Kitchen, garage, work shop, patio. Check monthly
Smoke detectors / Carbon monoxide detectors work-Check twice a year

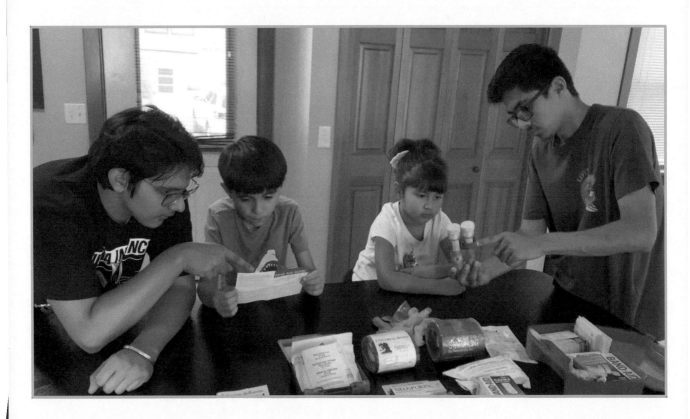

W – What should I do if…What about follow up care???

Talk it out. Play the "What If" game. What should I do if… this happens…?
What if someone gets cut on a knife in the kitchen?
What if someone fell down some stairs?
What if someone ate berries, now they are having trouble swallowing?
What if someone jumps in the pool, but they cannot swim well?
What other questions can we ask?

What would you do if someone got stung by a bee?

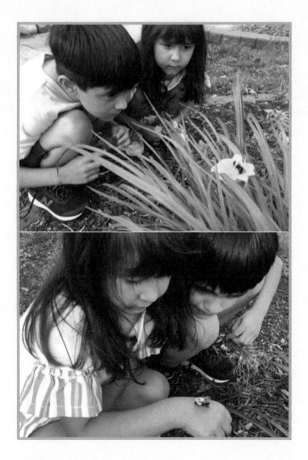

What would you do if someone were burned by grease?

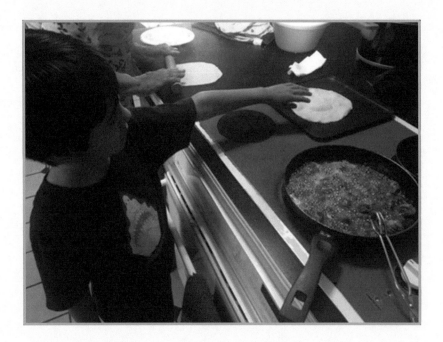

What would you do if someone hurt their leg?

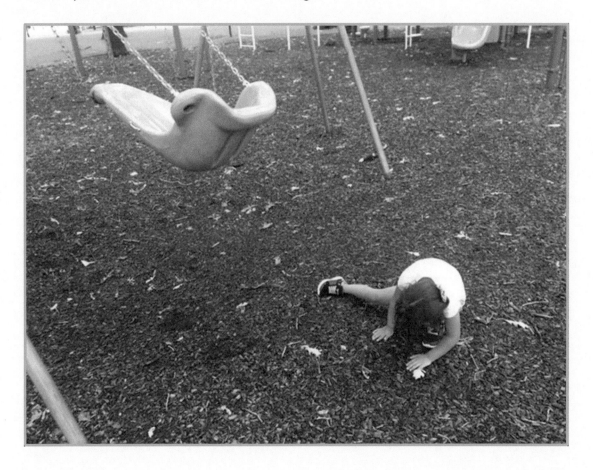

What would you do if someone were choking?

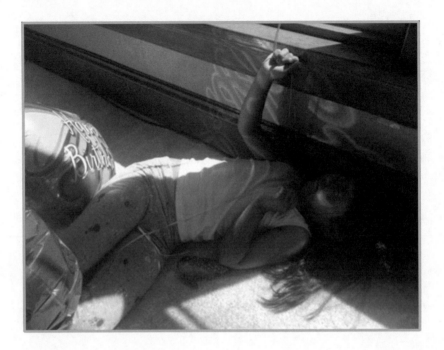

What about follow up care?

Do we need to change bandages? How often?
Do we need a tetanus shot? Where does the shot go?
Do we need to go back to see the doctor?

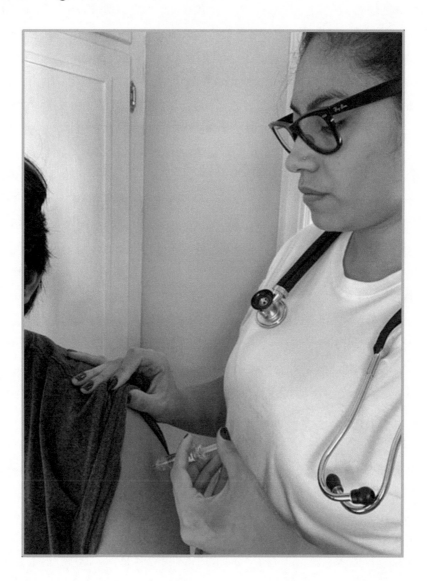

Scenario:

You and your friend are doing some archery practice at the park. An arrow bounces off of a tree and sticks in your friend's arm. What should you do?

C4-Stop shooting arrows. Now it is safe to help. You must first "C" the "Big Picture". You have 1 injured person. Check how bad is it bleeding? Do not remove the arrow if it is still stuck in the arm. Did you bring a first aid kit? Begin to **Control** the situation by telling your friend to sit down and be still. You can begin **Care** by holding the injured arm still. **Call** or yell for help. Is anyone around you who can help? Maybe they can use their cell phone to call 9-1-1. Or maybe they can run to the nearest house and ask for help? Can someone bring a first aid kit? If you are doing any activity where someone might get hurt, you should always have a first aid kit. Do you have a cell phone with you? If you have a cell phone, what do you say to the EMS dispatcher? Do you know where you are? "My name is _____. My friend and I are at the park on 4th St. We were shooting arrows and one got stuck in his arm. Please send help". Answer any questions they have for you. Is your friend talking or crying? Then the **Airway** is open! Is your friend talking or crying, then they are probably **Breathing**! If they are moving around, they probably have a pulse. What do you have to use for bandages? A lady across the street heard your cries for help and is bringing a first aid kit. She is using her cell phone to call 9-1-1. If you have gloves, put them on now. Hold direct pressure to the area and hold the arrow still to help their **Circulation** stay intact. Can your friend move their fingers? This is checking for a **Disability.** Your friend is probably very scared and in a lot of pain. Talk to them and tell them everything you are doing. If the arrow went through a shirt sleeve, cut the shirt sleeve around the arrow in such a way as to **Expose** the injury, but do not cause more pain or movement. Just be careful. Put on dressings or bandages now to help **Fix** the bleeding. Make a decision: Should you **Go** or Stay-Do you want to stay at the park and wait for the ambulance (recommended) or do you want to take your friend to the hospital? Do you know how to get to the hospital? How far is it? How are you going to get there? Walk, drive? Just make the best decision you can and go with that. Now you need to focus on keeping your friend from going into shock. **Halt** the shock now before it gets worse. Sit your friend down and make them comfortable. Elevate the legs. Do not let them eat or drink anything yet. If it is warm out, keep them cool. If it is cold out, warm them up. Gather **Information** on your friend for the doctor: How old is your friend? Does your friend have any allergies? Are they taking any medications, vitamins or supplements? Does your friend have any medical problems (other than the arrow in their arm)? When was the last time they ate or drink? What was it and how much of it? Check your friend's vital signs and **Jot** them down. How many times a minute are they breathing? How many times a minute is their heart beating (Pulse)? What does their skin look and feel like? Is it normal and warm? Or pale, sweaty/clammy and cool? Check your dressing to make sure the bleeding is controlled and the arrow isn't moving around. **Keep** everything you did right (stabilize the arrow) and keep everything you did tight (dressing and bandage). Has it been about ten minutes yet? If so, check your friend's vital signs again to see if they are improving. Now it is time to make a second call. Call the same emergency number and give them an update. Call your friend's parents. **Let** someone know how your friend is doing? When the medics arrive or when you get to the hospital (depending on your decision to Go or Stay) do a **Medical Hand-off**. Meaning you hand over your friend to a medical professional for more care. Now you can relax and catch your breath.

X – Expectations What do you expect to get out of your first aid training?

What do/can you expect from your loved ones?

> Expectations should be age appropriate
> Expectations should be realistic

Expect to improve every year

Y – Yearly Review

Update your emergency phone numbers
Update emergency meeting locations
Clear out the medicine cabinet
Practice first aid skills regularly. Each skill can usually be taught and practiced in 30 to 60 minutes.

Example:		
	January	Apply splints and dressing
	February	Burns: 1st, 2nd and 3rd degree
	March	Shock
	April	Hot weather injuries: dehydration, muscle cramps, exhaustion, heat stroke
	May	Choking and other breathing problems
	June	Bad cuts-Lacerations, avulsions and amputations
	July	Poison and chemical exposure
	August	CPR
	September	Moving an injured person based upon their injury
	October	Cold weather injuries: chilblain, frost nip, wind chill, hypothermia
	November	Foreign object in the eye
	December	Stroke: Act FAST- Face, Arms, Speech and Time it started

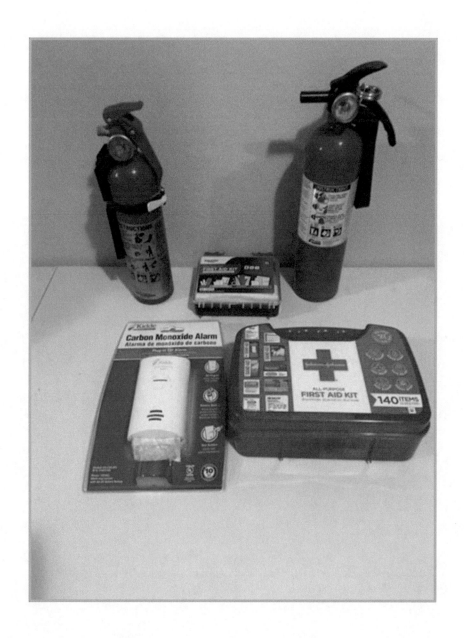

Z - Zombies If you see any zombies around it is not SAFE!!!...RUN!!!

Do not stay in a dangerous area to help others. The scene is not safe! Get everyone to a safe place before rendering care.

If you have to hastily move an injured person to safety, try to move them without causing more pain and injury.

Can you think of a situation where it is not safe to be there and help someone who may be injured?

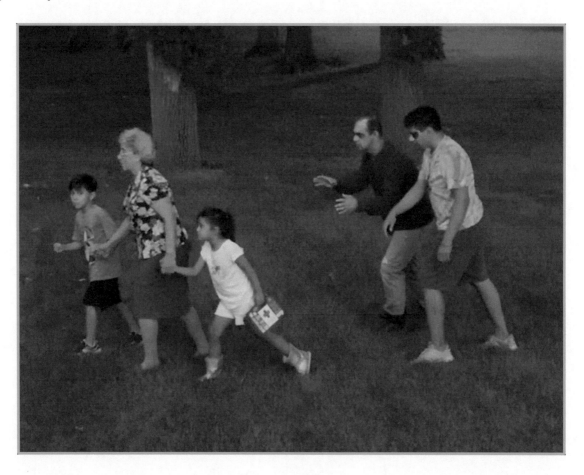

First Aid Kit Packing List – Remember to have multiple sizes, if they are available

Band-Aids	Tweezers	Antibiotic cream	Tylenol
Burn cream	Motrin	Hydrogen peroxide	Pepto Bismol
Eye Rinse	Antifungal cream	Tums	Calamine lotion
Scissors	CPR Mask	Tourniquet	Tape
Emergency blankets	First Aid Book	Gauze pads	Flashlight
Dressings	Thermometer	Roller gauze	BP Cuff
Ace wraps	Gloves	Co-ban	Hand Sanitizer
Ice/Heat packs	Hand Soap	Splints	Arm slings

What else would you add to your first aid kit?

_____

_____

_____

_____

The ABC's of First Aid

C4: Check, Call, Care and Control
Airway
Breathing
Circulation
Disability
Expose and Examine
Fix It
Go or Stay
Halt the Shock
Information Gathering
       SAMPL
       OPQRST
Jot the down the Vital Signs
       Breathing
       Pulse
       Skin
Keep things Right, Keep them Tight
Let others know what's going on
Medical Hand Off

Not going to happen to me
Open your mind, be Objective
P4: Plan, Prepare, Practice and Prevent
Question everything, especially pain
Recognize an emergency
Start doing something
Talk about things Before and After
Understand possible Hazards
Verify your stuff regularly
What should I do If...
Expectations
Yearly Review
Zombies mean RUN!!!

ABOUT THE AUTHOR

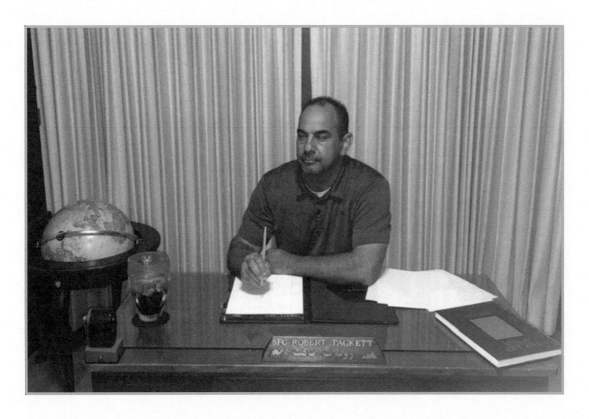

Robert Tackett has loved reading and writing his whole life. He is known as the family story teller who has told hundreds of stories to his kids, nieces and nephews and has promised to continue this family tradition through printed words. He has a wife, 5 children and a dog. A 23year Veteran, with 5 deployments as a Combat Medic under his belt has given him knowledge and experience known only to a few. It is time to get this information out to the world and hopefully empower the reader to be prepared in helping others.

Printed in the United States
By Bookmasters